Charm Her Socks Off: Creating Chemistry from Thin Air

By Patrick King

Dating and Image Coach at
www.PatrickKingConsulting.com

Charm Her Socks Off: Creating Chemistry from Thin Air
Introduction
The Biological Basis of Love

The Cuddle Hormone

Getting Head

The Nervous Sweats

Other Goodies

The Chemistry Principles
Chemistry Principle Number 1: Bold Dates Heighten Emotion.
Chemistry Principle Number 2: Spontaneity is King.
Chemistry Principle Number 3: Movement and Logistics are Essential.
Chemistry Principle Number 4: You are the CEO of the Interaction.
Chemistry Principle Number 5: The Activity is the Star.
Chemistry Principle Number 6: Interviews are for the Talking Heads.
Chemistry Principle Number 7: Eye Contact is Napalm.
Chemistry Principle Number 8: If Eye Contact is Napalm, Touch is Nuclear.
Chemistry Principle Number 9: Roll Out the Red Carpet… sometimes.
Chemistry Principle Number 10: She'll Appreciate Personalized Dates.
Chemistry Principle Number 11: She'll *Love* Boundary-Pushing Dates.

Introduction

Survey any of your friends and ask them what they're looking for in a significant other. Sure enough, you'll get a mix of the predictable following: great career, loving family, amazing parenting instincts, kind, considerate, matching hobbies, interesting, and attractive. The standard. We all know multiple people that fit these criteria, so does that mean that we're open to all of them as a life partner? Doubtful. (Though some of us undoubtedly take the shotgun approach.)

So the age-old question is raised: what makes us fall in love with one person versus another? All the slow jams in the world never seemed to be able to figure this out, but maybe that's because the answer is a bit of a nebulous construct. A spark. A click. A deep gut feeling of being drawn to someone. A certain *je ne sais quoi*. It's really not quantifiable outside of just deeming it *chemistry*.

Sharing the connection of chemistry with someone is one of the most wonderful feelings in the world. But for every 1 such connection we get, there are probably 4 other fizzled or friendzoned attempts that we'd rather not remember. Does *"I'm sorry... I just don't think of you that way"* sound familiar?

So the age-old question for most *men* ends up really being: how can I create that feeling of chemistry with any woman and make her fall for *me*?

In this book, I'm going to draw from my years of date coaching and use lessons from pop culture/TV to show you exactly how chemistry can be created with anyone.

"But Patrick, romance in pop culture/TV? It's all so fake and manufactured!"

A valid response, of course. But take The Bachelor, for instance. For those of you that are unfamiliar with it, the premise of the show is that there is one man who goes on dates with 25 amazingly attractive women. At the show's conclusion, which is a mere 6 weeks from the initial meeting, he invariably ends up proposing to one of them. That's a life-changing decision. If even $1/10^{th}$ of the emotional depth they develop on the show is real, that's still a lot of real chemistry and passion that cannot simply be explained away by the pressurized television and filming atmosphere.

I systematically analyzed these shows and broke down the commonalities of what drove chemistry and such intense feelings of love in short periods of time. Does being ridiculously handsome, being billed as The Bachelor, and a sense of competition amongst the other participants help? Perhaps. But beyond that, you'll be shocked at what really gets it done.

As it turns out, many of these elements are firmly rooted in the biological basis of love theory – in other words, what love does to our brains, bodies, and emotions. The rest just comes from smart planning and execution.

Dating shows exploit all of the above and veritably force-feed emotions into people. Anyone can do it, and I'll teach you how with my 20 Chemistry Principles designed to help you create chemistry... from thin air.

The Biological Basis of Love

It's helpful to first go over some of the physiological functions we're trying to take advantage of. The biology itself isn't the focus of this book, so I'm going to keep this section short and to the point.

For our purposes of cultivating attraction and chemistry, there are 3 main pathways at work, each of which I'll talk about briefly below. At their root, they are all simply biological functions which, with classical conditioning and association and clever planning, can be simulated and increased.

The Cuddle Hormone

You may have heard of this one. Oxytocin is known as the cuddle hormone because in general, it's released with more skin to skin contact you have with someone. It's also released in various social situations where people are relaxed and enjoying themselves. And when is it released the most? Directly after orgasm.

It causes feelings of trust and overall attachment to another person, and is said to be addictive. Your goal should obviously be to increase the release of oxytocin. If you've ever been accused of having no chemistry with someone, look no further than the lack of oxytocin.

Getting Head

Neurotransmitters are chemicals in the brain that are released in various ratios depending on the stimuli that the person is exposed to. There are 4 main ones, but the ones we are focusing on are dopamine and serotonin.

Dopamine is a neurotransmitter that is implicated in cocaine use. It is released by our favorite activities, anticipation, overcoming challenging situations, novel situations, and an increased heart rate. It provides intense rushes of euphoric pleasure... a phrase that accurately describes the rollercoaster of the early stages of any relationship.

Serotonin is implicated in many of the same causes and effects, but the main distinction is that when serotonin levels *drop*, people engage in obsessive thinking and ideation. Again, a phrase that accurately describes the dynamic of early relationships.

Your goal should be to increase the release of dopamine and decrease the release of serotonin.

The Nervous Sweats

Ever notice how fast your heart beats before you stand up to make a speech? How about right before you go in for that kiss? And further down the line, the butterflies and perma-smile that simply thinking about a lover can induce?

The release of epinephrine, or adrenaline, is the culprit here. Adrenaline is tied to your fight or flight nervous system, and technically serves to assist you in either battling a hungry bear or running for the nearest tree. Of course, these days it mostly serves to (in)conveniently remind us of situations we're uncomfortable or uncertain about, excited and thrilled about, and feel nervous and anxious about. Most importantly, it's a homing beacon to us that we're interested in someone.

We're all too familiar with the effects that adrenaline has on our body, and they're not generally beneficial, so why should your goal be to increase the release of adrenaline?

Human psychology dictates that when people are in any sort of emotional state, they seek justification for their condition. So if they are aroused, anxious, and thrilled with adrenaline, they'll attempt to mentally label the reason. In other words, if you get your date's heart racing on at least a semi-regular basis, she will attribute the causation to you, and chemistry is born.

Finally, when people are physiologically aroused and in a heightened mood due to adrenaline, they're going to be more positive and receptive in general.

Other Goodies

Pheromones remain somewhat of a physiological Bigfoot, but it cannot be denied that we simply prefer some people's scents to others. They have been hypothesized to be an invisible signal that mammals use to screen for genetic compatibility between potential mates, and a compatible pheromone may even sexually arouse the smeller.

What does this mean for you? Smell is a much greater part of chemistry and mating than most people realize. Act (and shower) accordingly.

Finally, endorphins: our biggest motivation for going to the gym. Endorphins are a neurotransmitter that is released after engaging in activities you enjoy, such as sex, exercise, singing, etc. It induces feelings of happiness and security. They function like an opioid, and are addictive by nature.

The Chemistry Principles

Now that we've nailed the basics of the biological basis for love, let's explore the Chemistry Principles that operate on them, among other factors.

The overarching theme and purpose of these Chemistry Principles is to take our biological and psychological functions, and turn them into actionable steps that the everyman can use to his advantage in any situation. Most importantly, I'll provide realistic examples that you can use *tonight*.

A Chemistry Principle will fall into 1 of 3 categories: Mindset, Interactions, and Communication. These are the 3 main elements that drive chemistry at any stage of a relationship, and therefore the most important for us to learn about.

The Mindset Chemistry Principles concern how you view yourself, and subsequently how that affects your interactions with women. They teach you how to be the type of man that a woman wants chemistry with.

The Interactions Chemistry Principles might be the biggest reason you bought this book. Through many specific examples, you'll see exactly what to do and where to take her to create a powerful bond with any woman. Your interactions and dates will never be the same.

The Communication Chemistry Principles are no less important than the other 2. The way you communicate is an offering that a woman may or may not accept. You'll learn how to use any form of communication to your advantage.

It's unfair to generalize an entire gender. Different Chemistry Principles will resonate with different women, but having all 20 in your belt will make you more reactive than the nuclei in nuclear fusion. (It's a book about chemistry, so I had to get one chemistry joke in!)

Gentlemen, let's learn how to hack a woman's emotions!

Chemistry Principle Number 1: Bold Dates Heighten Emotion.

This is Chemistry Principle number 1 for a reason. It's an all-encompassing general and more theoretical point that merits its own mention. Emotions that trigger the biology of love are powerful and your overall goal, and a bold date capitalizes on that. The bolder you can make your date, the more fondly she will think back on it. What woman doesn't want to be caught in the moment and swept off her feet?

It's also helpful to start the Chemistry Principles off here because it introduces the general mindset that you want to cultivate with women. Chemistry begins and ends with the spiking of emotional responses and bonds, so you want the operative emotions regarding your date to be shock, awe, wonderment, ecstasy, irrationality, joy, and above all, fun.

On dating shows, essentially every episode is punctuated by a helicopter or Amazon safari date. This is usually followed by an equally ridiculous activity, which leads to the woman barely being able to catch her breathe amidst the amazement. Her mind is so blown that she can't help but be entranced with the man who provided that experience.

Obviously, these are going to be impossible to replicate for a number of reasons, but there are some very doable alternatives and ways you can get the same reaction.

Remember that boldness is in the eye of the beholder. You need to be careful to ensure that she will actually enjoy what you're presenting to her, and that it will objectively wow her. Finally, though bold dates will inherently involve elements of physical activity and thrill, remember that bold dates can also be quieter. Bonus if it's a bold activity that you can take the lead in or teach her.

Examples:

1. Sky-diving
2. Bungee jumping
3. Whitewater rafting
4. Urban exploring at night
5. Sneaking into a closed building or park
6. Creating art together by finger or body painting
7. Riding ATVs in the desert
8. Jetski-ing
9. Renting a boat
10. Rock climbing
11. Getting ridiculed at a comedy show in the front row
12. Zip lining
13. Scavenger hunt with a list of clues personal to her
14. A shooting range

What she'll think: *This date is so crazy. He's so thoughtful, daring, and unique. I can't believe he thought of this. I can't wait to tell my friends!*

Chemistry Principle Number 2: Spontaneity is King.

"Hey, let's go into that store and adopt a cactus together!"

Spontaneity creates an effect where you appear like a laundry list of adjectives that women love: dominant, in control, adventurous, lighthearted, and fun. It's one of the best bang for your buck Chemistry Principles because of the emotional spikes involved.

Fortunately, as it turns out, spontaneity is mostly about appearances rather than true spontaneity. You wouldn't go into a big date without a plan. You'd have a plan with multiple options and paths, and your contingency plans would have contingency plans.

So the point here is to go into the date with a few "spontaneous" activities and interjections planned for later based on where you'll be and how it's going. Hell, sometimes your emergency plans can appear spontaneous if you pull it off.

Spontaneity is all about being (or appearing to be) willing to deviate from a set plan, and just letting loose and allowing fun to rule the day. You're in the moment and just enjoying her company, which will encourage her to do the same. It also instantly adds an element of novelty and excitement which can only work for you.

Indecision is the bane of spontaneity, so once you make a choice, stick with it. You should also take charge with any spontaneous detours, otherwise it can turn into a debate about what to do – the opposite of spontaneity and decidedly unattractive.

Practice tip: next time you hang out with your friends and walk by something interesting or funny, stop the group and take a picture with it. Really convince them, and don't just do it begrudgingly. This will condition you to the type of energy, body language, and excitement you must show for this Chemistry Principle to work.

Examples:

1. Movie-hopping
2. Eating different courses of a meal at different restaurants (appetizer, entrée, desert)
3. Date segmentation (see the next Chemistry Principle)
4. Climbing a tree in your path
5. Visiting the SPCA after driving by it
6. Buying a pet fish or plant for her, or for both of you
7. Last-minute anything
8. Going swimming in the beach after walking by it
9. Heads or tails decisions
10. Building a blanket fort in your apartment before watching a movie
11. Buying a disposable camera at a store and playing with it
12. Buying Nerf guns at a store
13. Chalking up a sidewalk

14. Experimenting with Mentos and diet Coke
15. Restaurant roulette

What she'll think: *He is so adventurous and creative! I can't believe we went all around the city tonight! Any date with him would be an absolute blast. He keeps me on my toes.*

Chemistry Principle Number 3: Movement and Logistics are Essential.

I explain this concept in one of my earlier books, so I've provided a short excerpt on it:

Plan the date in *segments* with natural ending points, which will allow you to bail early if you so wish. But if you like her and the feeling is mutual, then you can go proceed with the subsequent segment in your logistics plan, which you have arranged before the date. Do *not* tell her about the segments beforehand, as the idea is to make them seem spontaneous and fun in the name of spending more time with her.

This is an easy process. You've clearly already set up an activity that she agreed to for your initial date, so now it's time to do a little bit of support research. Before you go on your date, make sure you have the following easily accessible in your head:

1. What are 2 nearby <u>venues</u> you can go to after the initial date activity? *Bar, tapas restaurant, lounge, your place, a park with swings, a scenic view, etc.*
2. What are 2 nearby actual <u>activities</u> you can do after the initial date activity? *Karaoke, a walk/stroll, scenic view with a bottle of wine, billiards, bowling, biking, etc.*

If the first segment went well, proceed to the next. And so on. For an optimal date, I would recommend trying to complete 3 segments total. It keeps things moving, helps conversation, makes you seem knowledgeable and spontaneous, and creates more opportunity for flirting. It's also a great barometer into how she feels about you – if she keeps agreeing to go onto your next date segment, it's usually a very telling sign. Other things to plan for include:

3. Proximity to public transport and your apartment?
4. How familiar are you with the area? Get familiar!
5. Are you likely to run into people you know while out? In most cases, this is a plus.
6. Do you know the owners of any establishments? This is a major plus.
7. Can you showcase any skills or talents during any of the activities? For example, if you can sing, subtly suggest karaoke.

What she'll think: *That date felt like 3 full dates, and they were all great. I really got to know him and it never got slow or lagged. He really knows this area, and I was having such a ball.*

Chemistry Principle Number 4: You are the CEO of the Interaction.

Even if you're dating a woman who is a high-powered CEO, chances are that she doesn't want to be in control of your relationship. In fact, it's a good bet that she wants the exact opposite. There are exceptions to the rule, but many (if not most) women are completely fine satisfying the gender role of wanting to be taken care of.

It's hard to do that if she's making all the decisions and directing your interactions. So be the dominant man that she wants to sweep her off her feet. If you act that way, you'll project the confidence and masculinity and she desires. And just as importantly, the dominant man doesn't stay mired in insecurity.

On the surface level, some might call it chivalry, but that's a different mindset completely. Here, you are taking control of the interaction simply because you are the type of man to do so, not out of respect or deference to her.

This means that indecision is one of the most unattractive traits possible. The following type of exchange is strictly forbidden:

"What do you want to do/eat/see next?"
"I don't know, what do you want to do? I don't care."

So it's up to you to take control and plan the entire date with segmentation and backup options. You will lead the date through your segments. You will take care of the directions and not ask her to look up the address. You will provide a blanket, umbrella, or gloves just in case she needs them. You will deal with the bill (not necessarily paying) and address any issues that arise with the date itself. You will deal with the transportation. You will lead her through crowds. You will introduce her to the chef of the restaurant. I think you get it.

If you lead, she will take notice and follow suit. Most importantly, she'll respect you and your capabilities, which can write a one-way ticket away from the friend zone.

Practice tip: plan the next outing for you and your friends. Take care of all the planning details, the hiccups, dealing with waiters, splitting the check, renting the home, and controlling the guest list. This will let you know exactly what's needed for such an event (or date), and will give you experience and confidence in your abilities to take control. It will also make you more comfortable with potential confrontation when you have to fix or remedy a situation on a date.

However, note that there is a canyon of distinction between taking charge of the interaction and being one of the guys that will carry her purse for her. Take care of her, but don't cater to her. I like to utilize what I call the *groan test* here. If you can tell your male friends about something you did for her and their reaction is *groaning*, then you are probably catering to her too much.

What she'll think: *Wow, he took care of everything. He makes me feel safe and taken care of. He's a man's man, and I see him as my equal. I have to step up my game.*

Chemistry Principle Number 5: The Activity is the Star.

I touch on this in other books, but I have a strong opinion on what constitutes a good and a bad date. My opinion on the worst date of all? Dates composed of simply sitting and talking. Of course, this points to a dinner or lunch date. Many situations call for an exception, but as a general rule, I would only do a meal on a date as part of a date segment, or as a spontaneous act.

My reasoning is that this inevitably forces people into interview mode, which is a wholly inorganic way of conversation.

"So you know Doug?" "Yeah, we went to school together!"
"Oh cool." "So you know Brittney then?"
"Nope." "Oh, I see."

And so on. Think about how you started getting to know your best friends. It was almost certainly through a shared activity or interest, where you happened to converse naturally in the context of that activity or interest. There was little to no pressure to talk, which makes conversation flow more smoothly, organically, and tends to avoid the interview questions that plague many dates.

The solution to avoid an interview is an activity that takes the front stage of the date, which will decrease the pressure on continual conversation and let you two converse as nature intended. When the focus of a conversation is not the other person, the focus will be on having fun, comfort, rapport, and chemistry.

The activity still has to leave room for conversation though, so it can't be an overly loud, active, or public (in the sense that there will be many other people to interact with) activity. Activity dates are also extremely easy to tie into in-games, which I address later in Chemistry Principle Number 16.

Examples:

1. Mini-golf
2. Driving range
3. Cooking class
4. Cooking dinner together
5. Gardening
6. Hiking
7. Biking
8. Trivia nights
9. Painting class
10. Canoeing
11. Working out together
12. Building picture frames
13. Karaoke bar or private karaoke room
14. Painting pictures of each other with crayons
15. Bowling
16. Billiards
17. Playing with fake tattoos
18. Chalking up a sidewalk

19. Making terrariums
20. Go-kart racing

What she'll think: *That date was SO fun, and the conversation was so easy. He's such a great guy and I really felt like we got to know each other well. No awkward pauses!*

Chemistry Principle Number 6: Interviews are for the Talking Heads.

A talking head is an interview a TV character has with an interviewer off camera where they provide commentary about their thoughts and feelings. A date that is not.

Conversation is the cornerstone to any date, and really, relationship. You can have the boldest, most exciting date, but if your conversation lags and you can't effectively make conversation, any chemistry you've created will quickly fade and you'll be a two-date wonder at best. (Well, three-date wonder if you're rich.)

The most commonplace way that a conversation drags is when it turns into a job interview. See earlier for an example. It's characterized by jumping from topic to topic, staying on a surface level with all topics, and fishing for superficial commonalities that might not even be there.

We do this all the time at cocktail parties with people we are just meeting and anticipate talking to only for that night. Isn't that the only reason you ask Juan where he's from, or where he went to college?

But for a date, you've got to dig deeper and really strive to make a connection. The way to do this is not apparent to most people, so here are a few helpful guidelines.

1. A recent 2013 study showed that on a first date, both men and women had a better time when the focus of the conversation was on the woman. What does this mean for you? People like to talk about themselves, especially to people who show genuine interest in them. Be that person, so keep the focus on her, and don't dominate the conversation.
2. Don't jump from topic to topic. Ask "why" and "how" questions to dig deeper on the current one.
3. Avoid heavy topics such as religion and politics. If you get on those topics, don't judge or debate her.
4. Learn to have *great* reactions. For instance, when to laugh, roll your eyes, smile, gasp, and so on.
5. Don't fight breaks or silences in conversation. Let them happen and embrace the ensuing tension. Scrambling to fill a silence usually comes off as unconfident.
6. Don't rely on close-ended "who, what, when, and where" questions.
7. Instead of asking questions at all, first share about yourself and your stories, observations, and daily struggles. "I had the craziest day today…"
8. Learn what active listening is and use it.
9. Focus on commonalities that involve feelings, outlooks, and hobbies, not superficial ones like geography and mutual friends.

Practice tip: invite a friend over for dinner. Make it your goal to find out absolutely everything about your friend, and *talk as little as possible* except for digging questions. Try to hear their best and worst stories.

You'll find out how to create a line of questioning about topics you previously had no idea about, and which questions and tones are comfortable for you to use.

What she'll think: *I felt like we had known each other for years! He's so charming, and genuinely interested in getting to know me. I felt so comfortable and secure with him.*

Chemistry Principle Number 7: Eye Contact is Napalm.

What's that saying, that eyes are the window to the soul? Similarly, the eye contact you use is the window to your *masculinity*. The way you use eye contact is going to tell a woman how confident you are, how you feel about her, how interested you are in her, and whether you're an insecure or dominant man. Typically, the more the better, and this is an area where I highly suggest people fake it 'til they make it.

For practice, try making eye contact with strangers on the street. Once you lock eyes, don't pull away immediately. They likely will break first, and you'll be surprised at how empowering and confident it makes you feel. Now apply this feeling to your interactions with women, and you'll understand just what you've been missing out on.

Practice tip: next time you go outside, put sunglasses on and try making eye contact with strangers. Now that you can stare with impunity, you'll notice how many people completely avoid eye contact, and how many simply break it nervously after a quick glance even though they can't see your eyes.

However, don't stare at her like a moth at a lightbulb, and remember that there are times when the lack of eye contact is also potent. Imagine how you'd feel if someone's eyes started darting around behind you while you were talking. Were you talking too much, is she bored, or am I being boring or too weird... how can I get her eye contact back?

Eye contact, like much body language, can make points very succinctly if done correctly. The lack of eye contact doesn't necessarily have to indicate anxiety, it can also show boredom which can be powerful.

What she'll think: *I love the way he makes and holds eye contact with me. It really connects us. He's so confident and doesn't shy away from me. His gaze gives me goosebumps.*

Chemistry Principle Number 8: If Eye Contact is Napalm, Touch is Nuclear.

Friends don't kiss each other, friends don't put their arms around their friend's waists, and friends don't hold each other's hands. So if you want to be more than a friend, shouldn't you make an effort to do those things sooner rather than later?

Here's a dirty little secret about the friend zone. You're only going to end up there if a woman is simply not attracted to you physically or if you repulse her otherwise. If you don't fall into either of those categories, and you smartly utilize touch and some of the other Chemistry Principles, you will always be in the hunt.

Touch is perhaps the bedrock of the biological basis of love theory. Skin to skin contact literally causes the release of hormones and hearts to race. That intoxicating rush when you get close enough to smell someone's hair or brush fingertips? Oh yeah.

It also has the beneficial side effect of planting a mental seed and making them think about you in a sexual manner. After that thought enters their mind, it's just going to make them want more next time. Finally, a man who isn't afraid to touch knows what he wants and possesses confidence. Notice the running theme of confidence so far?

There are so many potential pitfalls here that I will just implore you to adhere to the following guidelines:

1. Less is more. If you only give her a little bit, she'll feel teased and want much more.
2. Is she still hanging out with you and laughing at your bad jokes? That's as good as a green light as you are going to get.
3. Don't let the first date pass without touch.
4. Don't ask her for permission.
5. In many cases, it is easier to touch from the side. Facing each other straight-on is more likely to create and violate a personal bubble, whether she realizes it or not.
6. Set the tone early on that you are a touchy person. If you aren't, learn to be.
7. Read her response like a flowchart. If she seems comfortable, escalate to more touching. Note that instead of verbally asking whether she wants to hug, hold hands, or even kiss, you're essentially asking her physically by doing it and moving forward. This is a much stronger and more confident move.

Examples:

1. Touching the small of her back while walking next to or behind her
2. Playfully hip-bumping or pushing her while walking
3. High-fiving
4. Pulling her legs on top of yours while you sit next to her

5. Playing with her hair while sitting next to her
6. Pretending to read her palm
7. Pulling her close by her belt loops or neck in a loud environment so you can hear each other
8. Grabbing her hand if you're rushing
9. Offering to show your new talent of massage
10. Playfully flexing your muscles and comparing to hers
11. Buttoning/zipping up her jacket for her
12. Trapping her under a blanket by wrapping her like a burrito
13. Lifting and throwing her into the air if she says something particularly funny or agreeable
14. Pretending to pull and hold her back before crossing a street
15. Helping her put on her coat
16. Scooting close to her and putting your arm around her while looking at a menu together

As you can see, most of these are much more subtle ways of touch that will allow you to gauge her reaction and determine whether you can move to the next step. Everyone knows how to kiss and put their arms around someone, but the subtle and flirty methods are much harder to learn and essentially pave the way for bigger gestures.

Practice tip: try some of the examples on your female friends. There's a 99.9% chance that they will have absolutely no problem with most of them. You'll learn that females don't mind touch, and indeed may crave it, which is a powerful realization. You'll also learn to push your boundaries, and become comfortable with being a more touch person, which is almost perceived as confident.

What she'll think: *I liked the way he touched me. He was flirty and subtle, and didn't go overboard or make me uncomfortable. I left wanting more! I hope he tries to kiss me next time.*

Chemistry Principle Number 9: Roll Out the Red Carpet... sometimes.

It never fails. Every season, the Bachelor will surprise a woman with a ludicrous date like being in the Broadway production of Lion King, and she is sent into mad giggles of "Are you *serious*?" I would probably giggle too.

But for those of us who don't have Broadway producers on speed dial, there are still steps you can take to roll out the red carpet for a woman, and put a special touch on a date that will make her feel special and highly desired. This Chemistry Principle is not about spending a certain amount of money, rather about demonstrating your thoughtfulness and effort in how you treat a woman.

If you can pull off a red carpet gesture in public, that's another bonus. If a woman likes flowers, she'll *love* getting them in front of others, especially other women, even if they are all strangers.

However, this is a Principle that is often approached the wrong way. There's a thin line between putting a personal touch on a date that shows that you put some special effort in, and pandering to her and spoiling her like a chump might. Hence the qualifier "sometimes," which is to say that you want to be unpredictable in showing her special attention, which will allow you to keep surprising her time after time.

Psychological studies have proven that inconsistent rewards yield the most anticipation and greatest subsequent satisfaction, so be the guy that makes her want more.

Another pitfall is a red carpet gesture that falls short, or isn't altogether that special like a generic red rose. It's certainly positive, once again the *groan test* rears its ugly head. If you tell a female friend about your proposed gesture and her reaction is a big fat *groan*, then your gesture simply falls short.

Finally, this is a chance to show her that you have the ability (or the appearance of) to pull some strings and make things happen. Power, or the illusion of power, is always a bonus.

Examples:

1. Getting a custom menu at a restaurant (most things custom, really)
2. Being greeted by a restaurant's chef
3. Being greeted by a ballplayer at a game
4. Backstage/VIP anything
5. Requesting a special song to come on the speakers
6. Hijacking the PA system to make an announcement
7. Having the restaurant staff sing for her
8. Throw up a website/blog dedicated to an inside joke you have with her (this is surprisingly easy and cheap if you use Wordpress and GoDaddy)

9. Spelling out a message for her with Christmas lights around her neighborhood
10. Getting a four string quartet to play during dinner
11. Scavenger hunt with clues personal to her
12. Organizing a surprise party for her with her friends
13. Cooking her a 3 course dinner

The common thread here is that they are things not necessarily done by you, but by third parties that you orchestrate. Gestures that come through other channels just seem more significant because it implies, as mentioned, power. This is precisely the reason why singing grams are a thing.

What she'll think: *He really pulled out the stops for me. He knows how to treat women, and he'll definitely treat me right. And so sweet of him!*

Chemistry Principle Number 10: She'll Appreciate Personalized Dates.

This is a Chemistry Principle that seems like common sense, but I like to leave as little to chance as possible. She's just going to have a better time, and each of the other Principles will work better, if you indulge her and take her on a date that involves something she enjoys. Duh.

This is meant to show that you have listened to her and put extra thought into putting together a date that is tailored, unique, and personal to her. You're also able to make her enjoy of one of passions or interests in a new and novel way, which is valuable. The idea is to incorporate her interests into a fun date for both of you.

Note that this does not mean to pander to her, to pretend that you like the same things she does, or to spoil her. Don't make it a gesture just for the sake of acknowledging one of her interests, because then it becomes all too obvious that you are just doing it for the brownie points.

Examples:

1. If she likes dogs drop by the SPCA or donate to them in her name
2. If she likes football take her to a local high school game and act like teenagers

3. If she likes cooking take an exotic cooking class together or do Iron Chef-esque challenges
4. If she likes cars pay a garage to give her a lesson on changing her oil (or teach her yourself!)
5. If she likes running take her to a trainer to get her stride analyzed
6. If she likes singing take her to a karaoke bar or open mic night
7. If she likes fine dining, hire a chef to come cook for you two at home
8. If she likes hiking take her to the market to make trail mix for your upcoming hike

These all tend to work better as surprises. Note that these are not dates where the activity she enjoys is the focus (which would be pandering), they tend to be educational for the activity in question.

Practice tip: take out a sheet of paper and write down 10 things she likes. If she hasn't told you 10 things, find out from what she owns, buys, eats, where she goes, etc. Then write 3 *activities* for each item that involves the item she likes. Like above, if she likes dogs: visit the SPCA, sit on a bench overlooking a dog park, or take a coffee break outside of a pet groomer's office.

What she'll think: *I was so surprised! He really understands me and managed to make it so fun for both of us. He is a great listener and is super thoughtful.*

Chemistry Principle Number 11: She'll *Love* Boundary-Pushing Dates.

Ever hear of the foxhole friendship, sometimes known as the boot camp bond? It's the type of bond that is formed by going through hardships and adversity together, and is used mostly in the context of war and soldiers for obvious reasons.

But lesser and different forms of the foxhole friendship exist in every walk of life. For example, even if you don't know them very well, an undeniable bond exists between teammates after grueling workouts, teammates after winning a hard-fought championship, neighbors under a tyrannical landlord, and co-workers under a Dilbert-esque boss. The common thread here isn't that they are *negative* events, rather that they are *superlative* events.

They can be the craz*iest*, cool*est*, hard*est*, weird*est*, funn*iest*, *worst*, *most* thrilling or confusing events, and as long as it's something you can laugh and talk about afterwards. It forms a mini-version of the foxhole friendship and brings you two closer instantly because it's a world that literally no one else can understand and that she only shares with you.

Engaging in a superlative activity is also a great way to demonstrate your vulnerability, and to show that you just want to have fun and don't care what others think (point of clarification: you can feel free to choose things that make you look terrible, but *not* humorless or mean-spirited).

So how can you take advantage of this bond? As the Chemistry Principle states, we can use boundary-pushing dates to foster the foxhole friendship. Just make sure that you're not completely crossing her boundaries or violating Chemistry Principle Number 10 (by doing something she honestly just hates).

Examples:

1. An actual boot camp class
2. Confronting fears (like scary movies, heights, the dark, public speaking, snakes, balloons, etc.)
3. Paintball
4. A grueling race
5. Taking a walking tour that is 3 miles longer than you thought, and in weather 15 degrees hotter than you thought it would be
6. Seeing a truly terrible movie
7. Being served by the most rude waiter in the world
8. Something you're both terrible at so you can laugh together
9. Something you're both great at and can compete at or against
10. Any class (the less you know, the better)
11. Learning to ride bikes if you both can't
12. A painfully early hike to see a sunrise
13. Playing catch in the rain on a muddy field

The two of you have to match in your perception of the date. You both have to think it was a superlative activity, or there is no foxhole friendship, and no shared bond.

What she'll think: *We got through it together! I feel so close to him after sharing it with only him. He can make any situation better. I'm going to smile every time I think about it and him.*

Chemistry Principle Number 12: Unique Should be a Given.

Unique dates have been the goal for guys since the word was invented. If not unique in itself, at least a unique location, activity, or event. Everyone wants to stand out, and flashing some of your obscure expertise is a natural way to do so. And of course, no one wants to do the same thing ad nauseam.

Our inclination towards uniqueness is because we know that it almost always generates positive reactions. We also instinctually know that the absence of anything unique is boredom. A unique date is always a plus in the grand scheme of creating chemistry, and gives us a higher floor and ceiling to start with – low risk and even higher rewards.

This is the Chemistry Principle that probably needs the least explaining, and where the examples are most important. This Chemistry Principle also ties in nicely with a few others, because it gives you a shared experience that will presumably make her excited and is easily bold and conversational.

Examples:

1. Geocaching
2. Riding Segways like tourists
3. A scavenger hunt around the apartment
4. Night hikes

5. The circus
6. $1 store craft projects
7. Hand or body painting
8. Urban exploration
9. Drunk Jenga
10. Making costumes for each other based on a movie you watched together
11. Watching airplanes takeoff near the airport
12. Iron Chef-style cooking competitions
13. Cooking Ethiopian food or some other food you both have no idea about
14. Building pillow and blanket forts and declaring war on each other
15. Paddle-boating and feeding ducks at a local body of water
16. Going to a shooting range
17. Renting a scooter (moped) together
18. At-home wine tasting
19. Blind food tasting tests
20. No hands pie-eating contest

What she'll think: *This guy is not like the rest. I can't wait to tell my friends about this date and how creative and unique he is. There won't be a boring moment with him!*

Chemistry Principle Number 13: Your Life is a Series of (Mini) Stories.

A big part of my work as an image coach focuses on discovering what kind of image you want to cultivate to the world, then curating your experiences to project it. Finding the right stories and experiences from your life to inject into conversation is where this begins.

This falls right in with the other Communication Chemistry Principles. Stories are an inside view to your personality, emotions, passions. Learning those about you is the first step in allowing a woman to relate and feel connected to you, so it's imperative that you learn how to take a close-ended question and expand it to your advantage.

This is going to require you taking a mental survey of the aspects of yourself that you want to highlight, then and making sure that it's something that is objectively attractive. To make that distinction clear, it's the difference between being proud of your video game prowess and being proud of your new artwork. By absolutely no coincidence, many of the **SURCCHH** questions I present in my other books (namely, the *Did She Reply Yet?* Series) are great ways to utilize mini-stories and show positive aspects of your personality.

"So what do you do?"
"I'm a marketing executive. It's pretty cool!"

"Oh, nice."

Let's try again.

"So what do you do?"
"I'm a marketing executive. I deal mostly with clients... just last week we had a crazy client that threatened to send his bodyguards to our office! I definitely wish I dealt more with the creative side."
"Oh my God. Did he actually send them!?"

See how the second example contains so much more substance for her to connect with, to avoid interview mode, and make conversation flow more smoothly? The next natural step in the conversation above is to organically talk about the crazy client and other funny aspects of work, instead of awkwardly playing *"Now how about you?"*

I implore you to cue up similar mini stories (~3 sentences) for some of the most common conversation topics that will arise, such as:

1. Your occupation
2. Your week
3. Your upcoming weekend
4. Your hometown
5. Your hobbies
6. Your favorite music
7. Your passions
8. Your education
9. Your apartment/house
10. Your mutual friends
11. Your dating history

12. Your experience with the venue you're at
13. The weather
14. Your family
15. Your pet

As you can see from my example, don't just answer the question directly. Make it a mini story that can stand by itself. Again, check if they portray you to be what you want as your image. Just don't get too personal, negative, or controversial, and don't dominate the conversation.

What she'll think: *Conversation was so smooth with him, we could have talked all night. He's so interesting, and is quite the personality! He's like no other.*

Chemistry Principle Number 14: Love is Your Ultimate Goal...

In my experience as a professional dating and image coach, most people play "the game" wrong. To try to win a woman over, they use artificial means to decrease how much interest they show in her, in adherence to the general theory that people want things they can't have. Sure, don't smother a woman or text her 10 times a night, but I disagree with the tactics that most people use (the "3 day rule" among others). They end up causing misunderstandings, drama, and are generally an immature way of interacting.

Demonstrating your interest in a woman, and in a potential long-term relationship, is an essential component of chemistry. Studies have shown that women crave affirmation, and often only reciprocate their feelings when they have it. Done correctly, you will also pique her curiosity to the possibility and make her envision that future with you... And envisioning is the first step to reality.

So don't disguise your interest for her or make your intentions ambiguous. But make sure that you do it in a *subtle* and nonchalant way – indirectly, or offhand in some manner. The idea is to plant the seed for her to fixate on and overanalyze in her spare time, as people do.

I'll repeat the previous paragraph for emphasis. There's a thin line you must tread here. Don't make it a topic of conversation. Don't overdo it. Don't dwell on it.

Examples:

1. Bringing up date ideas for next week or month
2. Telling her you're excited or happy to see her
3. Talking about compatibility with her
4. Telling her you miss her
5. Use future-facing sentences like "When we do x…"
6. Mentioning that you're interested in settling down
7. Integrating her into your friend circle
8. "Adopting" a plant or fish together
9. Discussing near and long-term future goals
10. Telling her you like her

What she'll think: *How refreshing it is to see a guy that's straightforward. He doesn't mess around, and he's a guy that knows what he wants. He's genuine, and I know I can trust him not to hurt me.*

I realize this goes against many ingrained beliefs about attraction and "the game." But the reason this Chemistry Principle works is because when people are playing "the game," they are manipulating their *perceived overall availability*. However, your *perceived overall availability* depends on a number of factors, only one of which is your interest in her. The next Chemistry Principle will address the other factors, and exactly how you can demonstrate interest and still win "the game."

Chemistry Principle Number 15: But Independence Wins the Game.

As I began describing in the previous Chemistry Principle, the best way to play "the game" is not to use artificial means or rules to manipulate your perceived interest in her. I noted how in fact, this can often work against you, as it can foster drama and misunderstandings, and not take advantage of timing.

In actuality, your *perceived overall availability* is what allows people to play "the game" effectively, and it is comprised of many factors, only one of which is how much direct interest you show in her. Other factors impacting that include: how often you go out with other friends, how many hobbies you engage in, how many other girls you are dating, how busy your job is, any passions you pursue, and essentially any other priorities you might have that would limit your availability. How many times have you heard a woman talk about liking guys with passions and their own lives?

People want things and people they can't have because of the implied mental correlation between unavailability and value. This is, of course, why the rich and powerful have an inherent leg up in dating. So the best way to play "the game" is to engage in priorities that actually limit your overall availability. If you feel the need to artificially increase the perception of something, let it be about your *perceived overall availability* as opposed to flinging ambiguity about your intentions with her. This is the difference between ignoring her because you don't want her to feel your interest, and being so busy that she isn't always a top priority. It's also going to increase emotions like anticipation, eagerness, and longing for you.

This is the true root of the whole "women love assholes" rhetoric, as the less available you are to someone, the more attractive you become. In short, when you're engaged in something, you become engaging.

Loading up on other priorities has a lot of additional benefits. It firmly puts you in control of your life and schedule, and almost makes being needy and dependent impossible in general. Never will you put a woman on a pedestal again.

Unlike some of the other Chemistry Principles, there are no real pitfalls to watch out for here. If you take my advice to heart and really focus on developing yourself as an independent and social person, you're probably better off than you were before. Just make sure that you don't come off with a cocky air of *"I'm so busy, wherever shall I fit you into my schedule?"*

This is a good point to introduce exactly how you can escape the friendzone if you've been wallowing there for a while. Of course, it has to do with independence and playing the game the right way. The first step is to simply dis-engage from the object of your affection for weeks, if not months. Chances are that you won't miss her friendship very much... because being friends with someone really isn't the same as having a deep friendship. The second step is to just peak in your independence and personal development, so that when you re-engage, you are essentially a new, more attractive person that she hasn't yet experienced or turned down.

What she'll think: *There must be something about him. He's confident, he's got so many options, and really pursues his interest. He's got so much going on that I'm lucky to be with him.*

Chemistry Principle Number 16: Introduce In-Games Immediately.

At some point, no matter how charming you are, you will hit a conversation lull. It's natural, unpreventable, and simply a hallmark of meeting someone new. You've learned the basics about each other, but haven't quite transitioned into fully sharing about your daily lives. You're also still stuck in impressing mode, and not yet relaxed and completely comfortable around each other. Don't panic.

One of the great ways to deal with any type of conversation lull is to introduce an in-game. The great thing about in-games is that you can use them to break the ice and increase comfort and rapport within 10 minutes of meeting, but also combat lulls and spice things up 5 dates in.

So what's an in-game?

Examples:

1. People watching
2. Making up stories about the people around you
3. Spotting couples on their first date
4. Bets/races
5. Dares/challenges
6. Truth or dare
7. Playing for prizes from a dollar store
8. Scavenger hunts

9. Arm wrestling
10. Putting fake tattoos on each other
11. Hide and seek
12. Punchbug
13. Pretending to read her palm
14. Picture bingo
15. Role playing
16. Making eye contact before every drink
17. Assigning nicknames
18. Re-enacting movies
19. Composing haikus about people you see
20. Playing human bingo in public

Aside from breaking up silences and injecting some energy into your conversation, there are some powerful psychological effects here. Playing an in-game creates a mindset that is totally and completely focused on the other person. You will be the only thing occupying her mind for the duration of the game, either directly or indirectly.

She could be surrounded by people in a crowded mall, but only be thinking about and looking for you. This is going to bring you closer instantly, as it's something only the two of you have shared. In-games are also amazing natural segues into unique conversation topics and physical flirting.

In-games are almost always appropriate, but don't just run down a list of them. That will appear contrived and gimmicky and like you have nothing of substance to talk about. You have to be able to balance being silly as the in-game demands, but also switching back to serious and substantive when necessary. No one likes a guy that can't be serious; it reeks of immaturity and is just annoying.

In-games can also be surprisingly mentally draining, so don't keep them going for too long, or be too insistent on playing. Recognize the natural ending.

What she'll think: *He can make sitting around doing nothing fun! What a great conversationalist. We have so many inside jokes already, he's hilarious.*

Chemistry Principle Number 17: She's a Classy Lady.

It's important to put ourselves in a woman's shoes on a date once in a while. Yes, heels really do suck. But you'll also learn the inherent assumptions and concerns they operate on.

In *Did She Reply*, I told you that one of a woman's biggest early concerns while dating was for their safety, and that you needed to make them feel safe and comfortable. This is completely logical from her perspective, especially if you didn't know her before the date. Check your actions for creepiness and over aggressiveness – there's a bonus tip for you.

But this Chemistry Principle focuses on one of the next concerns they have after their safety: their reputation. Specifically, their reputation in regards to their propriety. In other words, she wants to be a proper, respectable woman, and not the girl sloppily making out at the bar.

How can you even influence that?

It's pretty simple, actually. Build comfort and flirt outrageously while you're in public, but don't escalate matters physically until you're in private with her. This is best illustrated through the inner female monologue.

What she'll think in public: *Why isn't he putting his arm around me or trying to kiss me? I want to get closer to him but don't want to make the first move in public, too many people are around.*

What she'll think in private: *FINALLY! I've been thinking about this all night. Ooh, this feels naughty...*

It's not that women don't want the same things men do. They're just conditioned by society to be more ashamed of wanting it, especially in public.

So imagine the interaction as a balloon. All the sexual tension that you've built through flirting in public keeps getting blown into the balloon, but you're not releasing any of it until you're in private. At that point, the balloon is bursting with the tension, and likely to explode. This is a good thing, as the balloon is likely to explode... all over you.

A bonus here is if you take advantage of push-pull psychology. For instance, you "pull" her into that alley after dinner to finally kiss her and let a little bit of air out of the balloon... followed by "pushing" her away by restraining yourself and not touching her at the bar. It's going to drive her wild and keep tension high.

Like all rules, this one is meant to be broken sometimes, like if you're getting some serious bedroom eyes at dinner.

Chemistry Principle Number 18: Be Dangerous.

The last time I shoplifted, I was 11, and it was a cookie from the local 7-11. I can't remember the type of cookie, the weather, or who I was with, but I do remember one thing: the feeling of heart-pounding exhilaration when I concealed the cookie in my baggy jeans and walked outside.

(I'm not condoning shoplifting on your dates.)

That feeling of exhilaration is universal, and is triggered when you engage in something that you're not supposed to be doing. It's a thrill, gets your adrenaline pumping, and ultimately, it's *dangerous*. The buzz of danger is a feeling you should embrace and take advantage of with your dates.

By breaking small, inconsequential, or just rarely enforced rules or laws, you position yourself to be thrilling, exciting, nonconformist, bold, brash, badass, rebellious, confident, brave, daring, and apathetic to what people think about you. That list of adjectives basically amounts to you being a bad boy, but well within reasonable limits. People, not only women, are inherently attracted to elements of danger and excitement.

(I'm not condoning that you break laws on your dates.)

Examples:

1. Moviehopping
2. Pretending it's your birthday at restaurants to get free food
3. Smuggling alcohol into a movie or concert
4. Sneaking in somewhere after hours
5. Pulling her across a (safe) street intersection before you are allowed to walk via the lights
6. Sneaking into a neighbor's pool
7. Taking shortcuts through private property or buildings
8. Climbing over a fence
9. Sneaking a flask into a bar or club
10. Taking sneaky pictures of other people in public
11. Exploring a venue's VIP areas
12. Skinny-dipping
13. Playing with fireworks (safely)
14. Hide and seek in an abandoned building
15. Sneaking into an alley for excessive PDA

What she'll think: *I can't believe we did that! This guy doesn't play by the rules, he does what he wants! So confident. He makes my heart pound faster, and I love it.*

You would hope it doesn't have to be said, but if you're committing a breaking and entering on a date, it's probably not the right tone to set. You also have to gauge how uptight or anxious your date gets, as more stressful types might combust from the pressure. You'll also want to stay away from actions that make you seem questionable like stealing, as opposed to thrilling.

<u>Practice tip</u>: be dangerous. Break a small, inconsequential, or just rarely enforced law. Notice how your heart is pounding, your hands are sweaty, and your voice is shaky. That's not a good look, so the more practice you get dealing with the physiological consequences, the more confident and badass you will appear when you do it on a date.

Chemistry Principle Number 19: Cultivate a Vacation Mindset.

Let's take a moment here to think about one of the greatest pleasures in life. No, not socks right out of a dryer on a cold day, though that is pretty damn special. I'm talking about hotel sex.

Why is hotel sex so amazing? There are a few reasons.

First, though the partner and act itself are familiar, the surroundings are new. Having sex in a new location is basically changing the act as much as possible without having a different partner. I don't think I have to get into why that's arousing. Second, novelty is a huge aphrodisiac and drives our need to experiment sexually. It's why we all have kinks and fetishes that we engage in – to spice things up and keep our sex lives fresh.

Third and most importantly, hotel sex is amazing because a vacation mindset is created. (Though the fact that hotel beds are almost always bigger than the one you have at home warrants an honorable mention.)

A vacation mindset is when you forget all the concerns of the drudgery of your daily life and just *let go*. People feel so removed from reality that the issues they would normally be worried about aren't even on their horizons. When people let go, they lose their inhibitions, and are far more open and receptive to whatever is presented to them. There's a certain "why not" attitude, and experimentation comes along with it. She'll not only be more open to eating that dish, but anything *you* have to offer.

Barring an actual vacation, how can you cultivate a vacation mindset?

Examples:

1. Take her to parts of town she isn't familiar with
2. Restrict access to her phone (in a playful way)
3. Avoid serious or negative topics
4. Don't bring up work
5. Do a walking tour of your city
6. Role play that you're on vacation
7. Talk about vacations
8. Do touristy things around town
9. Stay at a hotel
10. Take lots of pictures
11. Plan outings together
12. Make an itinerary together

The main objective is really to create a happy atmosphere that will allow her to put her guard down and freely experience everything about you. Get her so wrapped up in the experience that she just wants to keep it going.

So isolate what makes her guards go up, then skew as far away from them as possible, because on a vacation, there are no worries or fears. A final benefit here is that you'll be able to create a "just the two of us" foxhole friendship by virtue of experiencing it together.

What she'll think: *It's like being on a honeymoon when I'm with him! I never think about anything else, and he's swept me off my feet.*

Chemistry Principle Number 20: Communication is a Fickle Bitch.

Most of us don't have problems with communicating in person. In fact, that's the exposure we seek and welcome. But when we're not face to face with the objects of our affection, different dynamics arise that can dramatically change people's perceptions. You can be the smoothest cat in the world on a date, but if you over-text for a few days, you can be relegated to an afterthought.

Communication by phone or text is a tricky subject (fickle bitch), and there exists a very thin line between overdoing it and not demonstrating enough interest. I generally try not to give text advice because it's all extremely contextual and there are too many "what if" situations, but behold my 10 commandments that will at least keep you near that thin line.

1. You shall not send that final text. It feels great to have the last word in an exchange, rather than tentatively waiting to see if she decided to reply to you.
2. You shall send texts that are not dependent on a response from her.
3. You shall not wait hours to reply just for the sake of it. But you may match the timing she uses.
4. You shall abide by the "out loud" test. You better be able to read your texts out loud to a friend

without wanting to jump off of a bridge. This includes punctuation and emoticons.

5. You shall text or call only with a purpose, namely logistics and arranging dates. Keep it short, and end it before it lags.

6. You shall propose specific times and locations instead of just asking if she's free because it will shorten the conversation by at least 4 texts.

7. You shall make references to your past conversations and dates. Saying that something reminded you of her is a great icebreaker.

8. You shall keep your phone in your pocket during your dates. Check it in the bathroom only.

9. You shall follow up the morning after a date. Here's your formula: great to meet you + funny sentence about a topic of conversation last night.

10. You shall only leave a voicemail if you have something important or specific to say or ask.

Practice tip: examine your text conversation with your friends. What percentage consists of just arranging logistics, and what percentage consists of actual conversation? I'm betting the vast majority is the former. Also look at how you begin text conversations with your friends on different days. I'm betting that they are mostly started with funny interjections, personal to your relationship. Finally, look at the ratio of texts that you both send. I'm betting that it's relatively equal.

BONUS! – Avoiding the Dreaded "Creep" Label.

We all have someone in mind when that word comes up. Women use this term liberally. You probably can't even articulate exactly why he's been stuck with that label, but you just know that he's turned off many a woman, and women will avoid him like the plague when going out.

Let's analyze what women really mean when they label someone a creep, and make sure that you aren't embodying those traits.

Being a so-called creep is mostly a function of two shortcomings.

First, there is a genuine lack of self-awareness, where the creep simply does not realize that their actions can be perceived as too forward, awkward, or just plain threatening.

As an illustration, someone who lacks self-awareness would suggest an abandoned warehouse as a first date, having no clue that it would frighten the hell out of his unsuspecting date. As hyperbolic as that that would be for a first date, we can easily imagine someone making a joke about it and not realizing why it's frightening, can't we?

The creep is likely forward in their sexual intent with women, but in a socially awkward manner, which is threatening to women as they can't discern exactly how serious the creep is being. Such forwardness is also uncomfortable, because it's considered lewd or inappropriate in every day conversations. Women also don't know how to deflect the creep, because they don't know how he will react to normal social cues of rejection. Which leads me to the next point...

Second, they lack the interpersonal intelligence to pick up on the subtle (and sometimes not) cues that women send to indicate their lack of comfort or interest.

The creep just doesn't know how to take a hint. A woman an do everything short of saying "NO!" and the creep will either dismiss it or not realize the intent behind her actions... and even if she says "NO!" he might think she's joking or really saying "YES!"

Sometimes, it's an intentional lack of awareness, or a disturbing sense of entitlement. Whichever the case, not being able to take "no" for an answer can be anywhere from annoying at best, to giving off rape vibes at worst. Such persistence can be scary, and turns an innocent and awkward creep into a dangerous one.

So what does all this mean for you?

If you're in debate about whether something might be creepy... it probably is. View things from the context of a woman who is smaller than you, and wouldn't be able to overpower you physically. Learn to pick up social cues of disinterest, such as not responding to you, not questions you questions, trying to escape the conversation, or closed or avoidant body language and eye contact.

Conclusion

"You're just not my type."

After reading this book, you'll never hear any variation of the above again. The friend zone will never be familiar to you. Sexual tension will be a given.

We've cut to the core of what really makes one person have chemistry with another – and how you can be that person. You've seen how to tailor your approach (Mindset), actions (Interactions), and interactions (Communication) for maximum success and chemistry. Each and every one of my Chemistry Principles contains actionable steps that you can start today. So what are you waiting for?

Sincerely,

Patrick King
Dating and Image Coach
www.didshereply.com

P.S. If you enjoyed this book, please don't be shy and drop me a line, leave a review, or both! I love reading feedback, and reviews are the lifeblood of Kindle books, so they are always welcome and greatly appreciated.

Other books by Patrick King include:

Did She Reply Yet? The Gentleman's Guide to Owning Online Dating (OkCupid & Match Edition) http://www.amazon.com/gp/product/B00HESY42G

CHATTER: Small Talk, Charisma, and How to Talk to Anyone http://www.amazon.com/dp/B00J5HH2Y6

The Coffee Meets Bagel Handbook... for Men AND Women http://www.amazon.com/dp/B00ILATYZS

Cheat Sheet

Chemistry Principle Number 1: Bold Dates Heighten Emotion.
Select dates that tend to impress, outrage, or otherwise go over the top to maximize the emotional impact by your date.

Chemistry Principle Number 2: Spontaneity is King.
Plan out spontaneity by utilizing your surroundings and be willing to deviate from any set plans.

Chemistry Principle Number 3: Movement and Logistics are Essential.
Attempt to complete 3 date segments for maximum flirting, and make a plan for your location.

Chemistry Principle Number 4: You are the CEO of the Interaction.
Take control of the interaction not because you want to be chivalrous, but because you are a dominant and leader of a man.

Chemistry Principle Number 5: The Activity is the Star.
Plan dates with activities to avoid interview mode and keep an easy flow of conversation.

Chemistry Principle Number 6: Interviews are for the Talking Heads.
Avoid typical interview questions by delving deeply into topics and asking open-ended questions.

Chemistry Principle Number 7: Eye Contact is Napalm.
Expand your eye contact comfort zone.

Chemistry Principle Number 8: If Eye Contact is Napalm, Touch is Nuclear.
She will never tell you to straight up touch her, so begin with subtle touches and read her reactions like a flowchart.

Chemistry Principle Number 9: Roll Out the Red Carpet... sometimes.
Give her a special treat that shows your thoughtfulness from time to time unpredictably.

Chemistry Principle Number 10: She'll Appreciate Personalized Dates.
Show her something she loves in a new light.

Chemistry Principle Number 11: She'll Love Boundary-Pushing Dates.
Strive to experience a superlative date that you can bond over.

Chemistry Principle Number 12: Unique Should be a Given.
Unique dates are low risk and high reward situations.

Chemistry Principle Number 13: Your Life is a Series of (Mini) Stories.
Rehearse answers to common questions to project the image you want.

Chemistry Principle Number 14: Love is Your Ultimate Goal...
Showing your affection and interest is often a good idea, but you must do it subtly.

Chemistry Principle Number 15: But Independence Wins the Game.
Develop your perceived overall availability to make a woman chase you.

Chemistry Principle Number 16: Introduce In-Games Immediately.
Play in-games to icebreak and otherwise create a world that exists only for the two of you.

Chemistry Principle Number 17: She's a Classy Lady.
Don't force her to reject your physical advances based on her propriety, leave them for private.

Chemistry Principle Number 18: Be Dangerous.
Break a couple of unenforced laws to get the adrenaline pumping.

Chemistry Principle Number 19: Cultivate a Vacation Mindset.
Creating a carefree atmosphere will make her more receptive to you.

Chemistry Principle Number 20: Communication is a Fickle Bitch.
Maintain the illusion of busyness and control over text and phone.

Avoiding the Dreaded "Creep" Label.
View your actions from the perspective of a woman concerned for her safety, and watch for social cues of disinterest.

Made in the USA
San Bernardino, CA
10 October 2016